Not Broken
Picking up the Pieces After Pregnancy Loss

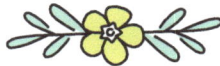

LORA SHAHINE, MD, FACOG
Illustrated by Sari Jack

Not Broken Illustrated: A Gift for Those Who Have Suffered Pregnancy Loss

ISBN: 978-0-9987146-4-6

Dedicated to my resilient and brave patients
who inspire me every day.
This is for you.

When you are expecting a child
You can feel hope, life, and dreams of what will be

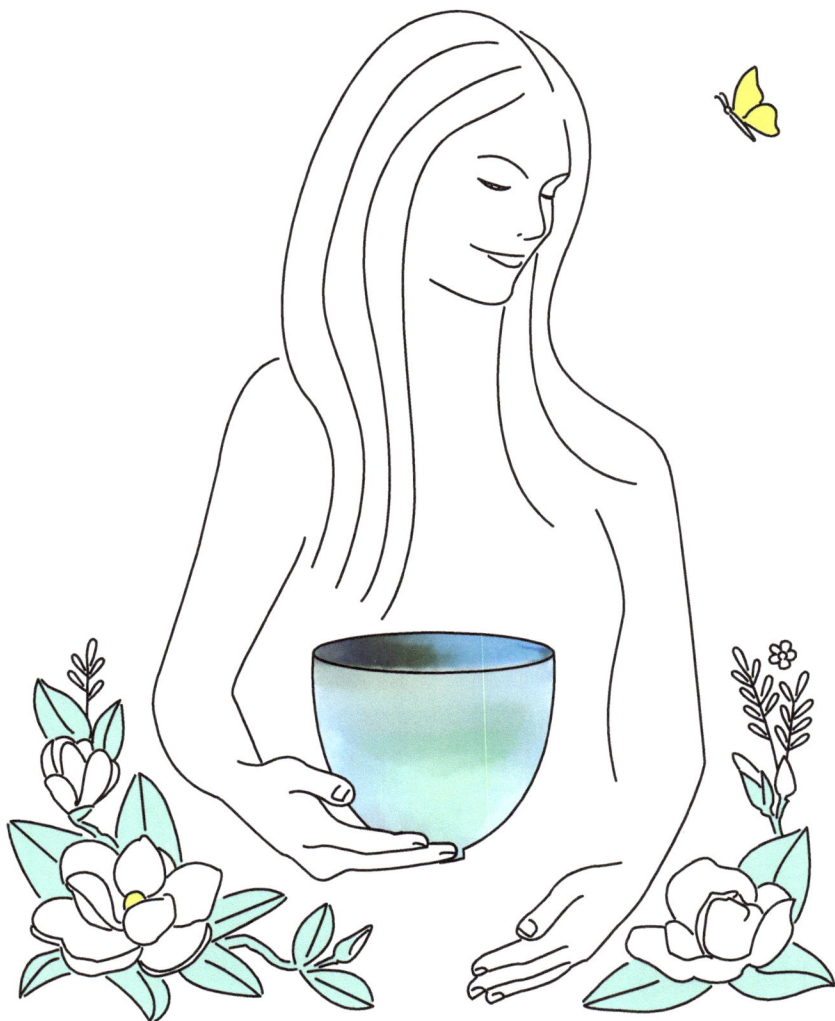

When you miscarry
No matter how far along
You can feel
Shattered

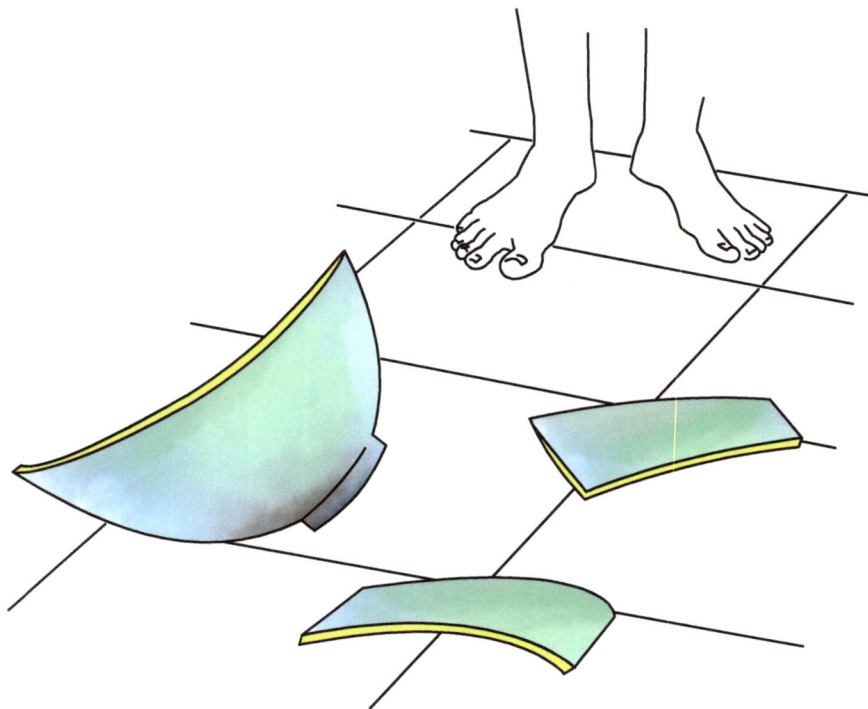

You can feel
Isolated

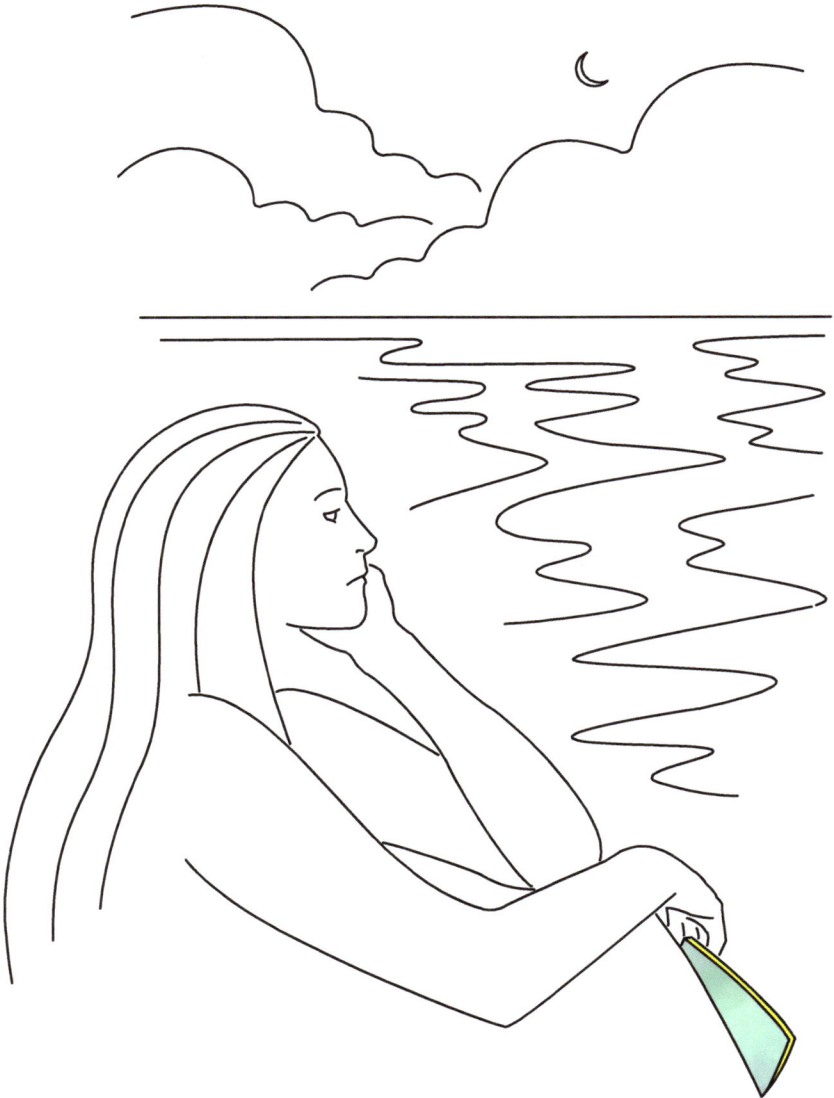

You can feel
Guilty
and Ashamed

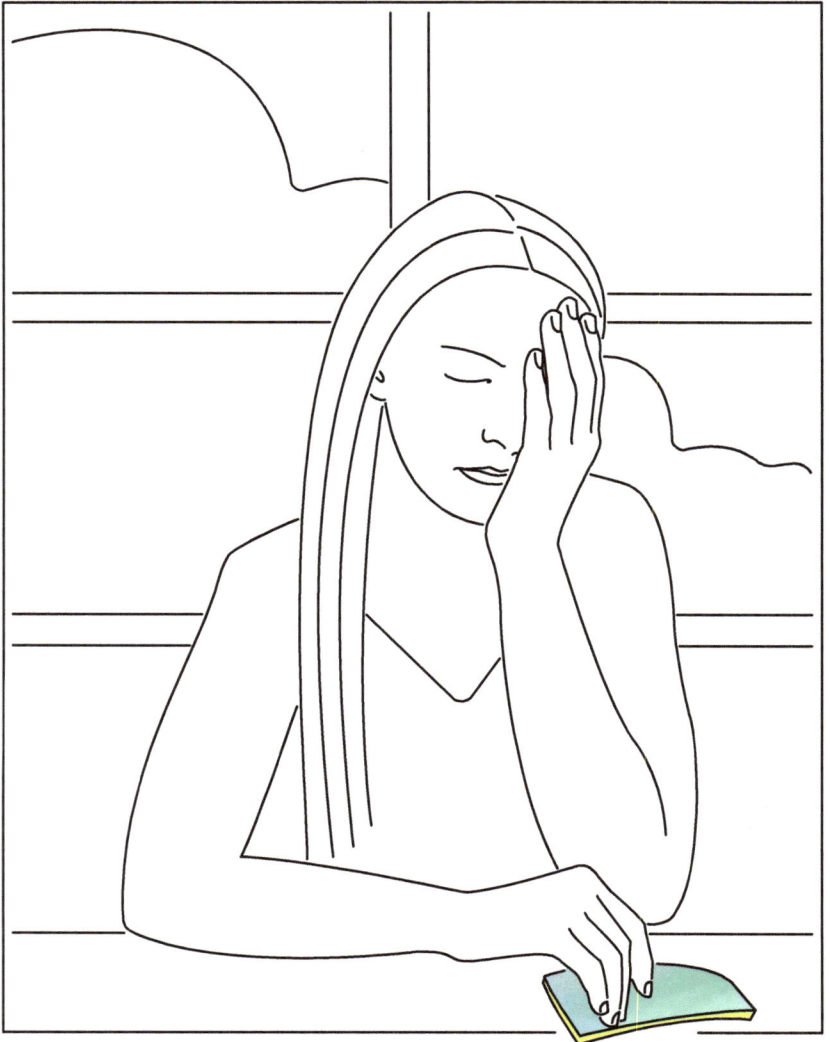

You can feel
Sad
and Angry

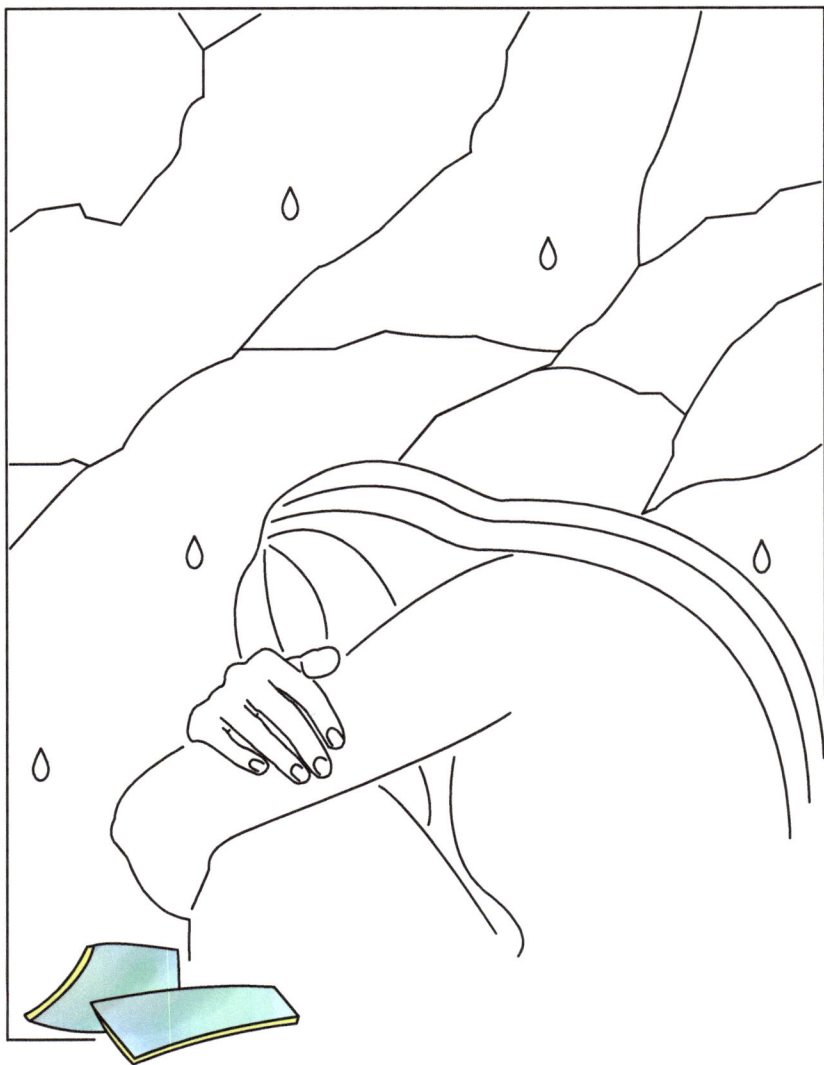

You need to know
It's not your fault
You did nothing wrong

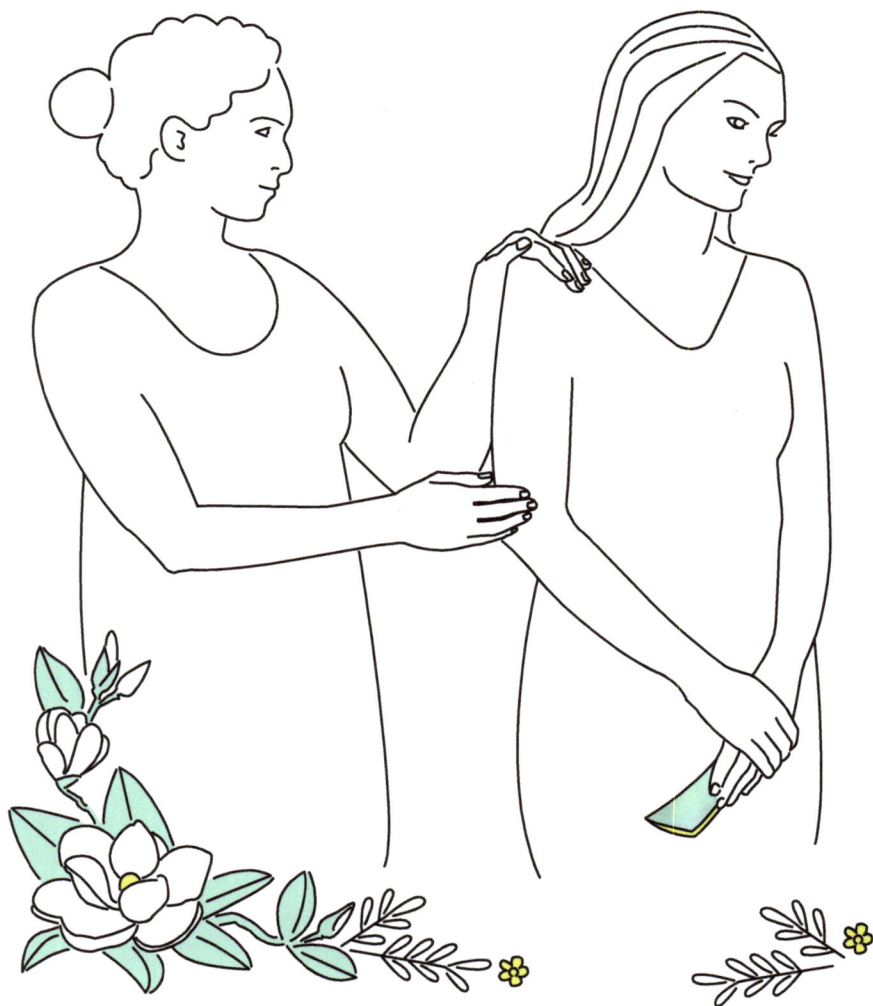

You need to know
You are not alone

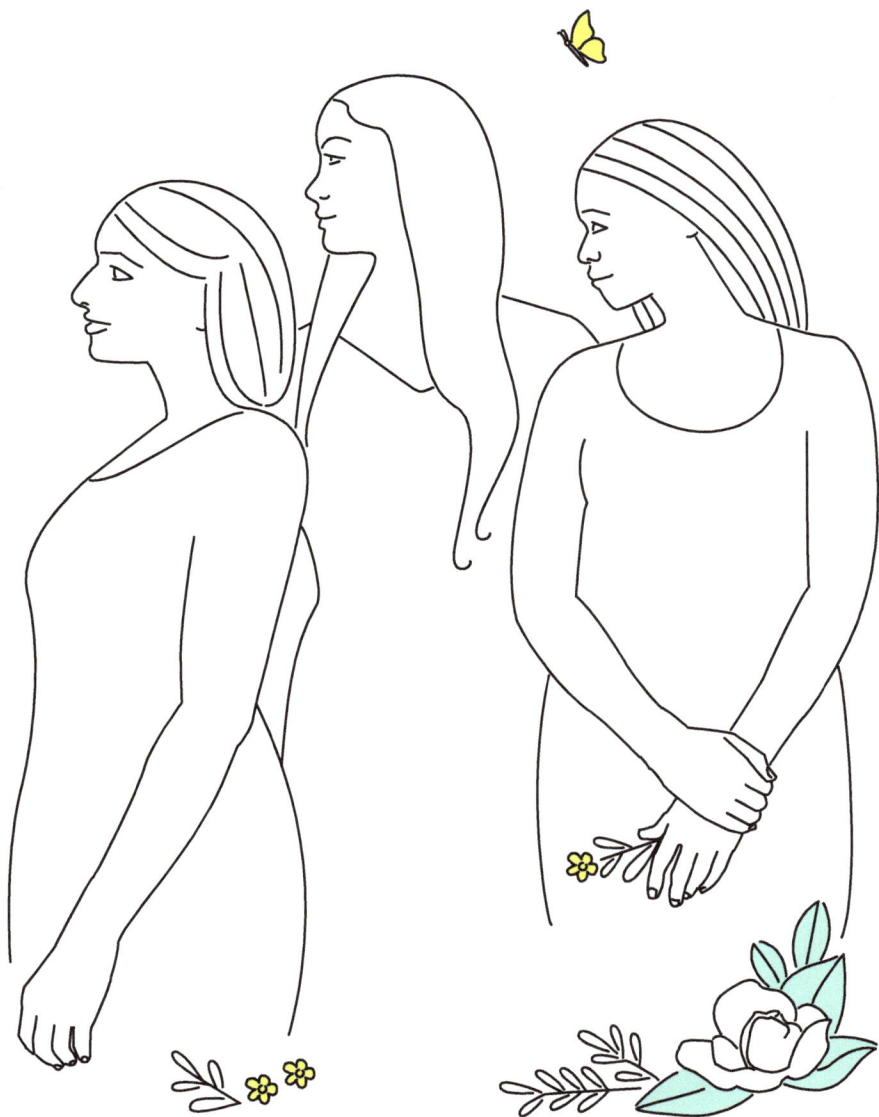

You can be
Strong

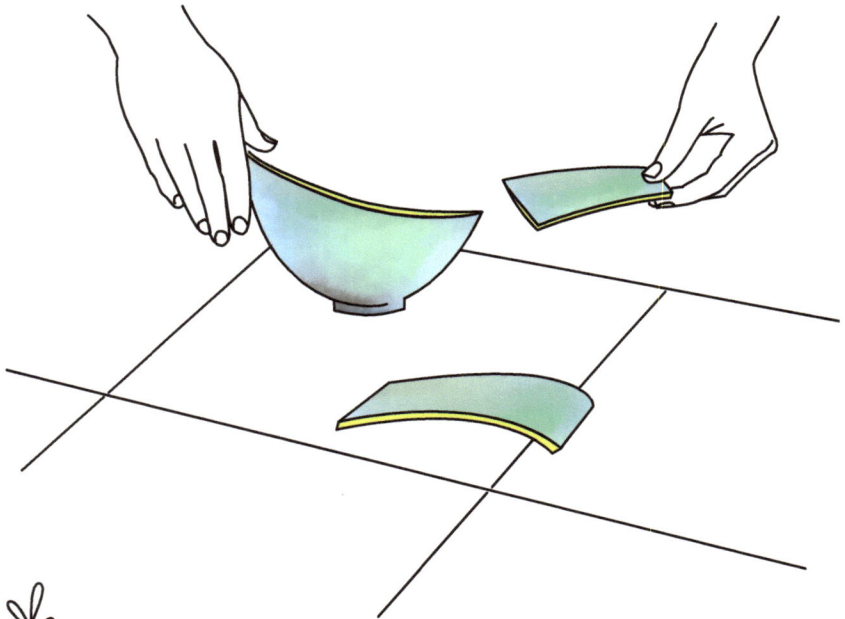

You can be
Brave

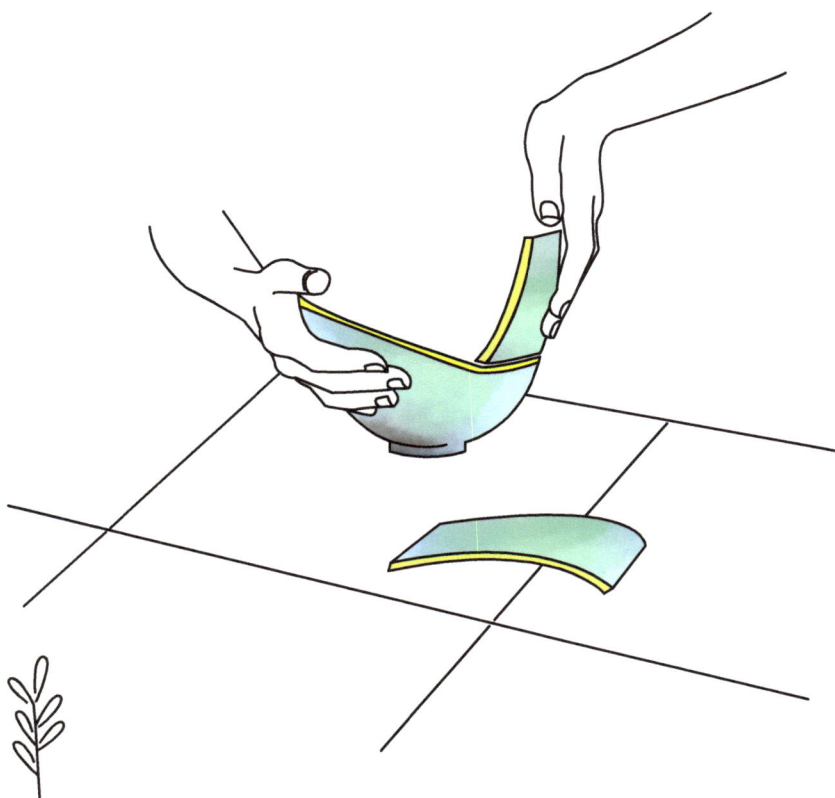

You can be
Resilient

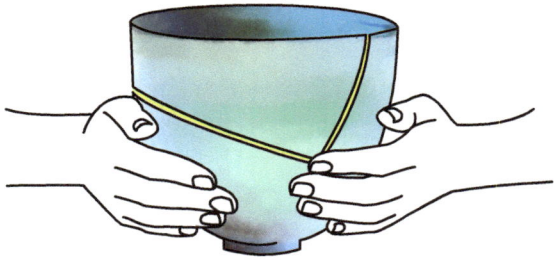

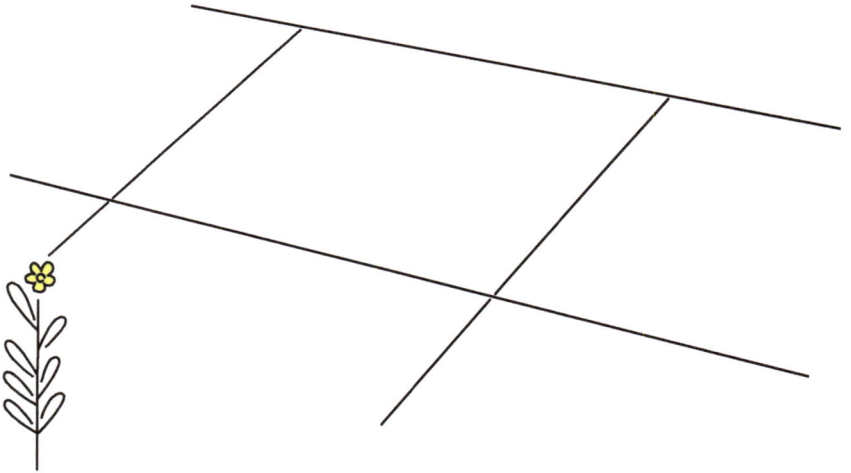

You are Not Broken

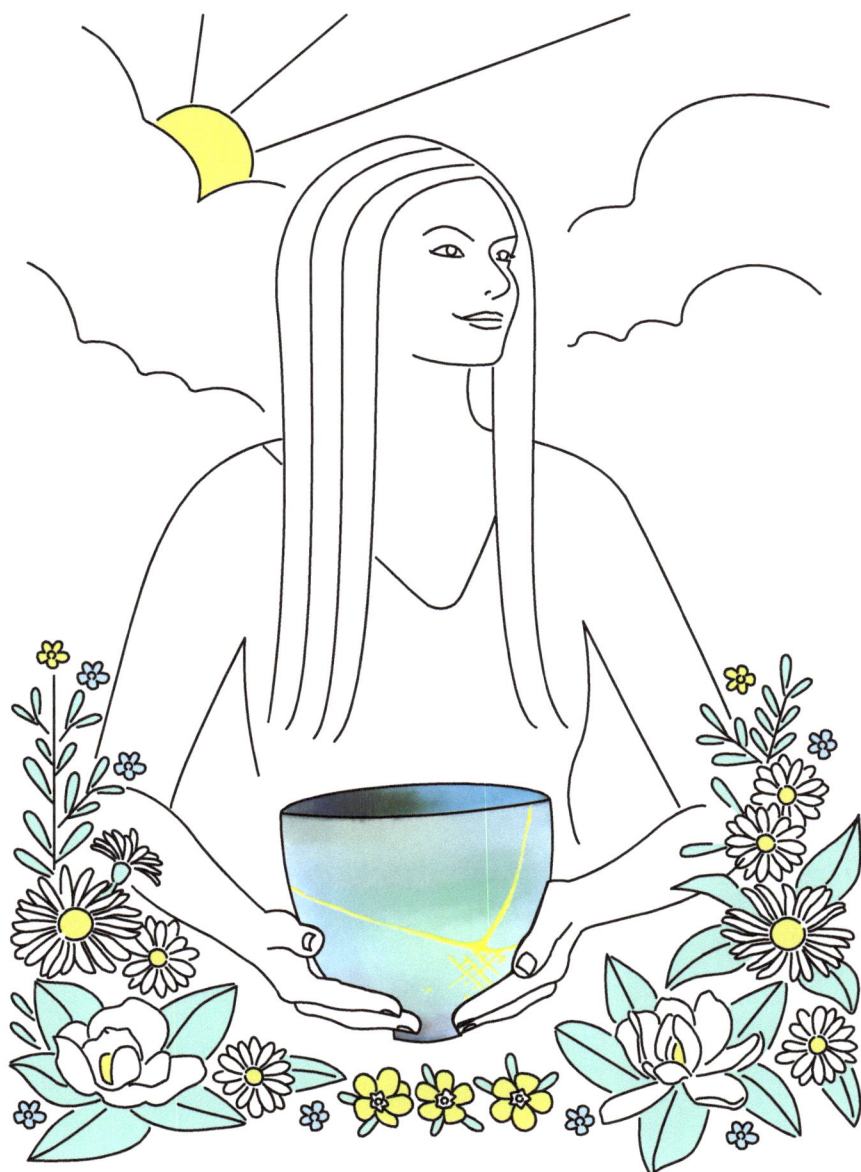

A Note from the Author

Miscarriage is common, but we still don't talk about it. Pregnancy loss is no one's fault, but it's surrounded by feelings of guilt, shame, and isolation. Some cultures honor, respect, and recognize the grief that surrounds miscarriage, but most do not. In Japan, it's customary to place a Jizo doll in cemeteries to protect over the souls of lost children, regardless of how far along the pregnancy loss occurred. In the United States and many other cultures, women are advised by medical providers not to share the news of a pregnancy until after the first trimester, 'just in case.' Most miscarriages occur in the first trimester, before women are showing, and with one in four pregnancies ending in miscarriage, most women suffer this loss in isolation far too often. Just when someone needs support the most, they are grieving alone.

Unfortunately, many of us do not know what to say and how to comfort someone who is grieving a pregnancy loss. Well-intended advice and personal stories can be inadvertently hurtful. Hearing "Everything happens for a reason" or "I know a woman who had 10 miscarriages before she had her baby" or "Maybe it was stress" can make a woman feel worse rather than supported.

I've written *Not Broken Illustrated: A Gift for Those Who Have Suffered Pregnancy Loss* to help comfort anyone healing after miscarriage. It's meant to be a source of hope and inspiration, and I imagine people sharing it with each other as a way to show support. In my humble experience, in the midst of grief, what we need is recognition of loss and the awareness that others care. Being supported when we need it most can be the greatest comfort.

Lora Shahine, MD, FACOG
Director of the Center for Recurrent Pregnancy Loss
at Pacific NW Fertility
Seattle, WA

The Emotional Impact of Miscarriage and Recurrent Pregnancy Loss

In my medical training, I learned about the diagnosis, treatment, and physical toll of miscarriage, but it's only been through years of caring for patients that I've realized the emotional toll and psychological impact of miscarriage.

I distinctly remember early in my fertility practice calling one of my patients with a positive pregnancy test and hearing a deep sigh followed by heavy silence on the other end of the phone. This was not the reaction of elation and happiness I usually got from my fertility patients who had been struggling to conceive.

After a moment, she said, "Thank you, Dr. Shahine, here we go again." I was stunned, and only after I hung up did it hit me like a ton of bricks– this test was the patient's fifth positive pregnancy test, and for her, this was just the beginning of the limbo, waiting, and anxiety until she knew whether this would be a successful pregnancy or not.

For her, this was only a beginning, and she had been down this road before with disappointment at the end. She would be on pins and needles until the next checkup – and the one after that and the one after that – and would only feel relief once she actually had a baby in her arms.

Studies have found symptoms of depression and anxiety and signs of post-traumatic stress disorder develop or become worse with miscarriage and recurrent pregnancy loss.[1] Patients report not only a grieving process, with all its stages, but an impact on feelings of guilt and doubts as to self-worth that can become worse with each loss.

Without support and understanding of the common causes of miscarriage, women especially begin to blame themselves for miscarriages. They blame their bodies, their stress, their diets. Without support and help, this can turn into self-blame and doubts of self-worth.

Men struggle with the psychological impact of miscarriage as well. They can feel angry, depressed, and helpless watching their partner go through miscarriage after miscarriage without knowing how to help or what to do.[2] Every person is different, but I've witnessed in my own practice many men extremely frustrated with a diagnosis of unexplained recurrent pregnancy loss – they want a problem they can fix, and leaving them with no clear answer is difficult.

Supportive care for patients with recurrent pregnancy loss is essential. Studies have shown decreased miscarriage rates for women who receive supportive care in the first trimester.[3] The authors of the studies cannot explain exactly why they see these results but argue that more contact with medical providers, emotional support through counseling, and comprehensive care should be considered for women with recurrent pregnancy loss.

There is no universal definition of supportive care for patients with recurrent pregnancy loss;[4] some describe it as counseling and emotional care, close monitoring in the first trimester with serial pregnancy hormone blood tests and ultrasounds, or both. Regardless of how one defines supportive care, all recurrent pregnancy loss patients are more likely to have signs and symptoms of depression and anxiety and should be offered support and wellness resources.

Support and Wellness Resources for Miscarriage

Emotional health is as important as physical health, and every person is unique, with different needs. Below is a list of support and wellness resources that I have found helpful with my patients

Counseling – One on one or couples counseling can be a wonderful resource for anyone dealing with the emotional struggles and grief surrounding miscarriage. The benefits of a counselor include privacy, individualized care, and an ongoing relationship with someone who can be supportive through future triggers and emotional ups and downs.

Patients often decline counseling at first – worried about cost, finding the time for appointments, and other concerns; but those who come back after connecting with the right counselor report feeling a sense of relief and security.

Take the time to find the right counselor – someone you connect with who seems empathetic to the roller coaster ride of struggling to complete your family.

Finding a counselor: If you have insurance coverage for counseling, start with your insurer's list to limit the financial burden of care. Ask for references from your health providers, friends, and online. When you call to make an appointment, ask if the counselor has experience with caring for people with infertility, miscarriage, and/or grief. Some counselors and therapists specialize in this area of care. If you do not feel a good connection with one counselor, don't waste your time and money – try someone new.

Support Groups – Some people enjoy the camaraderie they find when sharing their own experiences and listening to others share their personal struggles in a support group. Support groups specifically for recurrent pregnancy loss are less common, but support groups for infertility or infant and child loss support groups often welcome patients with recurrent pregnancy loss.

Finding a support group: Look online, ask your health provider and friends, or call local churches and hospitals. Churches often have support groups that do not require that you be a member of the church and are not always faith-based. If you do not share the same faith as a church with a support group – ask about joining – do not assume you can't. Some hospitals, especially women and children's hospitals, often have support groups available as well.

One very helpful national online resource for finding support is the National Infertility Association's website Resolve.org, which has a list of support groups across the United States. Resolve began in the 1970s and has become an excellent resource and advocacy group for infertility and miscarriage.

Mind Body Program – This is a program designed around the mind/body connection. Its foundation stems from observing biological responses (slowing heart rate, decreased blood pressure) with deep breathing and relaxation techniques at Harvard University in Boston in the early 1980s.

Dr. Alice Domar is the pioneer for studying and applying stress reduction techniques to help women with infertility. She runs programs through her Mind/Body Center in Boston, but other therapists and counselors run programs throughout the United States based on her model. The programs usually involve 8-10 week sessions of weekly meetings in which people learn stress reduction techniques and often share their experiences with others.

Meditation – The practice of meditation has become increasingly popular. Definitions differ, but in general, meditation is the practice of quieting the mind, relaxing, and bringing into focus a goal, a mantra, or a state of being calm. There are many resources for learning how to meditate, including books, online resources, and even apps for your smartphone that walk you through the process. Meditation can be intimidating, but give it a try. Be kind to yourself and try a little each day – it takes practice.

Mindfulness – Mindfulness is a practice of self-awareness and striving to be present in the moment. It is grounded in Buddhist meditation, but it is not strictly meditation. Mindfulness is being present, being aware of your body, your thoughts, your life in a single moment. It is taking time each day to stop, breathe, and be aware of sounds, feelings, and thoughts. It's a way to quiet the mind and reset, and it can be a useful stress reliever.

Mindfulness can be less intimidating than meditation for beginners. There are simple exercises that you can do quickly on your own to try it out. Look for resources online and several books written by Dr. Ellen Langer, social psychologist at Harvard University and 'mother of mindfulness.'

Yoga – Yoga is a group of physical, mental, and spiritual practices that originated in ancient India. Today, yoga is incredibly popular, and there are many different types of yoga practice, from slow, stretching, meditative yoga to hot, intense, club-music pumping yoga. Yoga for fertility has become popular, and many of my patients find yoga improves their physical mobility and decreases their stress.

If you have never tried yoga, it can be intimidating at first when the instructor calls out moves and positions you are not familiar with or you are stretching next to someone who can wrap their leg around their head twice. Watch a beginner's video online before your first class, find a studio with beginner's yoga, and forget the other people in the class – we all start somewhere! Don't use the excuse "I can't do yoga because I'm not flexible" because people do yoga to increase flexibility. Try it!

Self-Care – Self-care is taking good care of yourself, and it is an essential part of your overall wellness. In the everyday hustle of family, work, friend, and community commitments, it's easy to put our own needs last. Self-care means putting yourself and your needs first. Consider these tips:

1. Be kind to yourself.
2. Make sleep a priority.
3. Exercise, but give yourself a break from it when you need to.
4. Eat well – plan ahead and make healthy, well-balanced dietary choices.
5. Say 'No' to social engagements and extras at work if possible when you need a break.
6. Surround yourself with positive, supportive people.
7. Nurture your partnership – infertility and miscarriages are

extremely difficult on couples. You are in this together – be kind and supportive to each other.

8. Ask yourself, 'What am I going to do for myself today or this week?'

In Summary

Dealing with infertility and recurrent pregnancy loss have been compared to dealing with chronic disease and even cancer. Similar feelings of frustration, isolation, and questions like 'Why me?' surround these conditions, but the reactions from friends and the support provided can be different. As a society, we know what to do when someone gets cancer – we have meals to organize and flowers to send. But people suffering with recurrent pregnancy loss often suffer in silence.

Most miscarriages are in the first trimester, before people are physically showing pregnancy and before they announce it publicly. When miscarriages occur, women so often feel guilty in some way that they don't want to share with friends and family. Even worse, when people have the courage to share, they can find awkward responses from their support network about things they could do differently next time, which just makes them feel even more shame about how their body 'failed' them.

Find the support you need and take care of yourself through this journey!

References

1. Farren J, Jalmbrant M, Ameye L, Joash K, Mitchell-Jones N, Tapp S, Timmerman D, Bourne T. Post-traumatic stress, anxiety and depression following miscarriage or ectopic pregnancy: a prospective cohort study. BMJ Open 2016;6:e011864.

2. Kong GW, Chung TK, Lai BP, Lok IH. Gender comparison of psychological reaction after miscarriage-a 1-year longitudinal study. BJOG 2010;117:1211-9.

3. Liddell HS, Pattison NS, Zanderigo A. Recurrent miscarriage—outcome after supportive care in early pregnancy. Aust N Z J Obstet Gynaecol 1991;31:320-2.

4. Musters AM, Taminiau-Bloem EF, van den Boogaard E, van der Veen F, Goddijn M. Supportive care for women with unexplained recurrent miscarriage: patients' perspectives. Hum Reprod 2011;26:873-7.

About the Author

Dr. Lora Shahine is a board-certified reproductive endocrinologist practicing in Seattle, WA. She is the director of the Center for Recurrent Pregnancy Loss at Pacific NW Fertility, which opened in 2010 with the mission to care for patients, teach medical providers, and further research into the field of recurrent pregnancy loss. Dr. Shahine enjoys writing, and in addition to her own blog has authored two books, *Planting the Seeds of Pregnancy: An Integrative Guide to Fertility Care,* with Stephanie Gianarelli, LAc, and *Not Broken: An Approachable Guide to Miscarriage and Recurrent Pregnancy Loss.* Find more resources at lorashahine.com and connect @drlorashahine on Instagram, Facebook, and Twitter.

About the Cover

The image of the bowl throughout the book represents the Japanese art of kintsugi, in which broken pottery is repaired with gold-dusted lacquer. As a philosophy, kintsugi embraces the cracks in a mended object as a part of its history that should be highlighted, not hidden after repair. To me, this means there is beauty in our flaws, our grief, our experiences, both good and bad. We are not broken by our grief but made stronger, more resilient through our experiences.

Acknowledgements

Thank you to Sari Jack for her beautiful illustrations, Juli Douglas for the lovely image of the bowl, and Lucy Elenbaas for her editing talent!

Resources on Miscarriage and Support

Not Broken: An Approachable Guide to Miscarriage and Recurrent Pregnancy Loss – Dr. Shahine's book. A comprehensive, evidence-based but easy-to-read guide for understanding all aspects of miscarriage and recurrent pregnancy loss. She reviews testing, treatment options, controversies in care, Western vs. Eastern approaches to care, and the importance of paying attention to the emotional impact of miscarriage. Available in print at amazon.com and in electronic versions on Kindle and iBooks.

Lorashahine.com – Dr. Shahine's website with blog posts, book reviews, and many resources on infertility, miscarriage, and the emotional impact of both.

Resolve.org – A patient-centered and run website with information and links to support groups by zip code.

Asrm.org – The website of the United States reproductive endocrinology professional society, which has education materials for patients and providers regarding recurrent miscarriage.

Notes

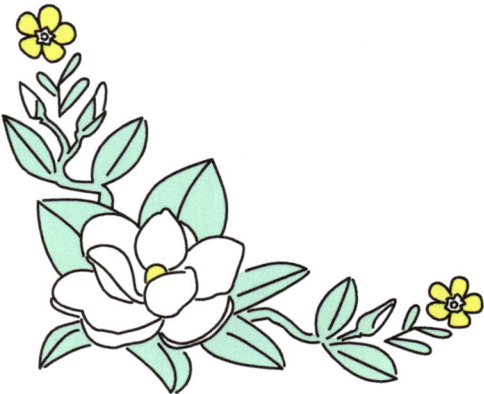

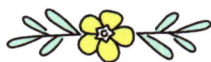

"We are all broken, that's how the light gets in."
–Ernest Hemingway

www.ingramcontent.com/pod-product-compliance
Lightning Source LLC
Chambersburg PA
CBHW041225270326
41933CB00006B/217